Ketogenic Diet For Beginners

The Ultimate Beginner's Ketogenic Diet Weight Loss Plan Guide For Men & Women

By *Louise Jiannes*

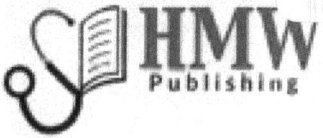

For more great books visit:

HMWPublishing.com

Download another book for Free

I want to thank you for purchasing this book and offer you another book (just as long and valuable as this book), "Health & Fitness Mistakes You Don't Know You're Making", completely free.

Visit the link below to signup and receive it:

www.hmwpublishing.com/gift

In this book, I will break down the most common health & fitness mistakes, you are probably committing right now, and I will reveal how you can easily get in the best shape of your life!

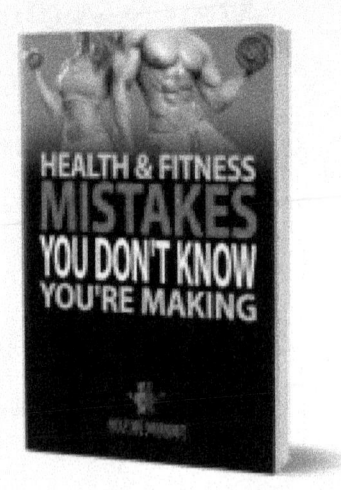

In addition to this valuable gift, you will also have an opportunity to get our new books for free, enter giveaways, and receive other valuable emails from me. Again, visit the link to sign up:

www.hmwpublishing.com/gift

TABLE OF CONTENTS

Introduction 1

Chapter 1 – What Is The Ketogenic Diet? 4

    What is the Ketogenic Diet All About? 4

    Why is the Ketogenic Diet so efficient? 6

Chapter 2 – Advantages Of The Ketogenic Diet 10

Chapter 3 – Disadvantages Of The Ketogenic Diet 17

    It Is Not an Actual Weight Loss 17

    Issues Maintaining the Low Carb Diet for A Longer Period of Time 18

    Reduction in Bone Mass and Density 19

    Constipation 21

    Hypoglycemia (Low Blood Sugar) 22

Chapter 4 – Ketogenic Diet Plan 23

    Setting-Up the Diet 24

    Weekend Carb Load 26

    How to Get Start with Ketogenic Diet? 29

Chapter 5 – Foods To Apply Ketosis Diet 32

    Fats and Oils 33

    Protein 35

    Vegetables 37

    Nuts and Seeds 37

    Beverages 39

    Sweeteners 40

Chapter 6 – Ketogenic Diet Mistakes and Tips **41**

    Increase the Intake of Protein 41
    Not Eating Enough Fat 41
    Not Eating Enough Sodium in Eating Regimen .. 42
    Exercises to conduct during your diet 43

Chapter 7 – Ketogenic Recipes **44**

    Snacks 44
    Drinks 44
        Peanut butter and Cacao Protein shake 46
    Breakfast 47
        Breakfast Meal #1 - Cinnamon Protein Waffles 47
        Breakfast Meal #2 - Ketogenic Low Carb Pancakes: 50
        Breakfast Meal #3 - Microwave Flax Muffins: 52
    Main Course 53
        #1 - Low Carb Pizza: 53
        #3 - Avocado Egg Salad: Ingredients 58

Final Words **60**

About the Co-Author **61**

Introduction

I want to thank you and congratulate you for purchasing the *"Ketogenic Diet for Beginners"* book.

This book contains proven steps and strategies on how to lose weight using a ketogenic diet and will provide you with everything you need to safely get started in the right direction including some delicious recipes to try!

You will also learn what exactly this diet is and how it works, the advantages of the ketogenic diet as well as some of the disadvantages (there are some). You will learn how to properly get started with this diet plan as well as learn which foods to apply the Ketosis diet. Lastly, you will uncover some of the most common mistakes as well as receive some helpful tips to make sure you don't fall in any of those pitfalls. Thanks again for purchasing this book!

Also, before you get started, I recommend you [joining our email newsletter](#) to receive updates on any upcoming new book releases or promotions. You can sign-up for free, and as a bonus, you will receive a free gift. Our *"Health & Fitness Mistakes You Don't Know You're Making"* book! This book has been written to demystify, expose the top do's and don'ts and to finally equip you with the information you need to get in the best shape of your life. Due to the overwhelming amount of mis-information and lies told by magazines and self-proclaimed "gurus", it's becoming harder and harder to get reliable information to get in shape. As opposed to having to go through dozens of biased, unreliable and un-trustworthy sources to get your health & fitness information. Everything you need to help you has been broken down in this book for you to easily follow and to immediately get results to achieve your desired fitness goals in the shortest amount of time.

Once again, to join our free email newsletter and to receive a free copy of this valuable book, please visit the link and signup now:

www.hmwpublishing.com/gift

Chapter 1 – What Is The Ketogenic Diet?

The Ketogenic diet also referred as Keto diet, low carb diet, and low carb high-fat diet is a low carb diet that produces ketones in the body. Ketones are the organic compounds that any human body has. With the help of ketones in the liver, a human body can produce energy.

What is the Ketogenic Diet All About?

Here's a brief history lesson, the Ketogenic eating diet was initiated in 1924 by Dr. Robert C. Atkins. A Ketogenic diet treatment was delivered right on time in the twentieth century to treat youngsters efficiently with refractory medication epilepsy. An immediate examination demonstrated that immersed fat is undesirable notwithstanding when a high-fat

Ketogenic eating routine is required, as in different medicines of uncontrolled epilepsy. A two week deliberately controlled inpatient study was conducted that demonstrated that a Ketogenic eating routine was valuable for the control of weight and blood glucose fixations in diabetic patients

In spite of being exceptionally viable in treating epilepsy, it dropped out of design because of the surge in new hostile to seizure medicines in 1940. The eating routine of this diet is high in fat, supplies adequate protein that is sufficiently required by a human body and is low in starches (carbohydrates). This blend changes the way vitality is utilized as a part of the body. Fat is changed over in the liver into unsaturated fats and ketone bodies. Another impact of conducting this diet is that it brings down glucose levels and enhances insulin resistance.

Glucose is the simplest atom for your body to change over and use as vitality so that it will pick over some other vitality source. Insulin is delivered to handle the glucose in your bloodstream, by taking it from the body. After the glucose is utilized as an essential vitality, your fats are not required and are in this way put away. Ordinarily, on a typical, higher sugar eats fewer carbs; the body will utilize glucose as the fundamental type of vitality to be picked during the process.

Why is the Ketogenic Diet so efficient?

The Ketogenic diet is one of the most effective diet plans that is being recommended by various doctors in today's world. The diet helps people lose weight and have control. The diet works so well because it ensures you maintain a low carb diet. Moreover, the amount of shedding of the weight depends upon the

BMI of one's body, activity levels and the kind of food that people are eating, but the estimate of losing weight by following this diet plan is maximum one month. That means that a human body starts losing weight of around 20 kilograms in the time duration of one month. The quickest approach to get into ketosis is to practice on an empty stomach, confine your sugar admission to 20g or less every day, and be watchful with your water consumption.

Initially, before the industrial revolution when humans were involved in hunting and gathering of food the issues about weight and health were quite low. People use to eat the food that was available to them by hunting, fishing and gathering food from nature. These foods did not include any starch as foods like pasta, rice and bread were not introduced until the industrial revolution. Therefore, carbohydrates in the human body were also low.

It started with the industrial revolution when a lot of development took place around the globe. Various factories began to appear, and they increased their operations in producing a significant amount of sugar and white flour. All this resulted in an increase in carbohydrate in the human body. This is the reason that in today's world people are more prone to obesity and other health-related issues. Countries like the USA that are considered one of the most developed nations of the world has been more inclined to this disease of obesity.

To eliminate this disease of weight gain and obesity various programs and diet plans have been introduced. All these methods have affected and helped people positively, and a Ketogenic diet is one of those weight loss plans recommended by various nutritionists. The Ketogenic diet is essential for people who are trying to lose weight, especially those facing substantial weight gains and are unable to shed pounds in a short span of time. Gaining weight results in various health problems and can endanger the lives of many humans. Therefore having a diet of low carbohydrates that would focus on reducing the glucose levels and enhancing insulin resistance is vital for most people.

Chapter 2 – Advantages Of The Ketogenic Diet

The Ketogenic diet is one of the most efficient and effective diet plans that contain low carb and it is beneficial in many ways to the human body. Since 2000, there have been various researches conducted in identifying the impacts of low carb diets. And in every study, the effects of low-carb diet was more positive than any other thing with which it is compared. Low carb diet does not only help humans to lose their weight, but it has also proved itself helpful in reducing and eliminating various risk factors that can be serious and harmful for a human body.

Since Ketogenic diet is a low carb diet, it does not stop an individual from eating something along with refraining from sugar-related food. Hence, this diet starts to kill the appetite of an individual. Many people are conscious about their weight; they try to reduce kilogram and maintain a balanced weight but to achieve their target they often had to stop eating. Eating less or eating nothing is something that is not possible for anyone as it leads to hunger and results in people giving up their diet plan. Therefore, an advantage of the Ketogenic diet is that a low carb diet allows an eventual reduction in the appetite as people shift their selves to low calorie based and protein related food rather than having food that results in weight gain.

Another advantage of a Ketogenic diet is that low carb food results in an instant reduction in the weight. People who reduced the carb level in their diets found themselves having a tremendous decrease in their weight. Hence, this food can be considered a most effective and efficient for people who want to shed pounds quickly. One reason for this is low-carb diets tend to dispose of overabundance water from the body.

Since they bring down insulin levels, the kidneys begin shedding abundance sodium, promoting fast weight reduction in the first week or two.

The Ketogenic diet also leads to increase in HDL that is high-density lipoprotein. HDL is good cholesterol. It diverts cholesterol from the body and to the liver, where it can be reused or discharged. It is understandable that the higher your levels of HDL, the lower your danger of heart diseases will be. One of the ideal approaches to building HDL levels is to eat fat, and low carb diet incorporates a tremendous amount of fat, which would result in an increase in High-density Lipoprotein and would save people from various heart diseases.

When an individual eats carbs, they are separated into basic sugars (generally glucose) in the digestive tract. From that point, they enter the circulation system and raise glucose levels. Since high blood sugars are lethal, the body reacts with a hormone called insulin, which advices the phones to bring the glucose into the phones and to begin smoldering or putting it away. For individuals who are solid, the rapid insulin reaction tends to minimize the glucose "spike" with a particular end goal to keep it from hurting them.

It is due to this reason many individual faces various issues such as insulin resistance. Insulin resistance implies that cells do not see the insulin and along these lines, it is harder for the body to bring the glucose into the phones. This can prompt an ailment called sort two diabetes when you do not emit enough insulin to bring down the glucose after suppers. This sickness is exceptionally normal today, burdening around 300 million individuals around the world. Therefore, the solution that various doctors in today's world recommend is a shift towards low carbohydrate diet as it leads to a reduction in insulin level and it would result in a decrease in blood sugar as well. There have been various studies conducted, and one of the studies stated that people suffering from type 2 diabetic 95.2% have experienced positive results and identified a reduction in their glucose within six months.

Blood pressure is one of the common phenomena experienced by a majority of the population across the globe. People suffer from high blood pressure and low blood pressure. Blood pressure itself encourages various diseases such as heart diseases, kidney failure or stroke and it can result in loss of life. Hence low carb diet is considered one of the effective tools for a reduction in blood pressure. And when people would experience a decline in blood pressure then chances of heart diseases, stroke or kidney failure also reduces.

Low-Carb Eating regimens are the best treatment known against Metabolic Disorder. Metabolic

Disorder is the name for a gathering of danger components that raises your risk of heart diseases and other wellbeing issues, for example, diabetes and stroke. There are various symptoms identified for this disease such as high triglycerides, Low HDL levels, and increase in blood sugar, an increase in blood pressure and increase in weight or fat near the stomach. Hence, with the introduction of the low-carb diet, all five symptoms can be reduced as an individual starts experiencing a reduction in their blood pressure level, in their weight and their HDL tends to increase and the person can live a healthy life.

The Ketogenic diet is more efficient when compared with a reduction in eating something or going for strict diet plans, as during that phase people start starving and end up in giving up the diet plan, and this leads to further health issues. Hence, Ketogenic diet encourages an individual to eat, but it should contain less carbohydrate, which ultimately improves the digestion system of an individual.

Chapter 3 – Disadvantages Of The Ketogenic Diet

Though there are tremendous advantages of introducing Ketogenic diet in one's daily routine as mentioned in the previous section such as high HDL, quick weight loss, lower heart diseases, and strokes, etc. there are adverse impacts that can affect an individual in opposite way as well. Some of the negative effects of Ketogenic diet are discussed below.

It Is Not an Actual Weight Loss

While going through the process of a Ketogenic diet, one loses weight quite frequently, but most of the weight that a person loses is the water that a human body possesses. And once your body enters ketosis, you likewise start to lose muscle, turns out to be to a significant degree exhausted, and, in the end, enter starvation mode. At that point, it turns out to be considerably harder to get into shape and lose weight.

The British Diabetes Association likewise calls attention to that ketosis is possibly hazardous, "as elevated amounts of ketones can make the blood acidic, a state known as ketoacidosis, which can prompt certain disease in a short space of time." Losing weight is good for one's health but relying solely on a Ketogenic diet can result in serious health issues as more heart issues are the outcome of this diet. Hence Ketogenic diet should only be conducted under the supervision and recommendation of a doctor.

Issues Maintaining the Low Carb Diet for A Longer Period of Time

Another disadvantage of performing Ketogenic diet is some individuals find it difficult to carry or sustain this, especially those who regularly attend social functions, go to school, or frequently go to restaurants. For example, a student who is following the Ketogenic diet and his or her peer eats high carb food in school, then he or she would also be tempting to have that kind of food. Hence, they would not be able to sustain their diet plan and end up in giving up their diet plan. Since carbohydrates provide an individual with most of the energy hence reducing sugar may cause reduction in the energy level of an individual. And the person tends to feel lazy, and might expect disturbed and frequent mood swings.

Reduction in Bone Mass and Density

Another negative impact of conducting Ketogenic diet is the decrease in the bones mass and its density in the long term. There have been various studies conducted, out of which one experimented on mice. During these experiment mice set on a fleeting

Ketogenic diet discovered a diminishing in bone-mass thickness and affected the mechanical properties of bones negatively. However, it needs to consider distinction in the middle of ketosis and the lifespan of the two unique species before accurate conclusions can be made. There have likewise been reports of diminished bone thickness in youngsters who maintain a Ketogenic diet for quite a while.

Be that as it may, a study on adults with a genetic issue called GLUT-1 lack disorder, who were kept up on a Ketogenic diet for over five years did not demonstrate any significant adverse consequences for bone mineral substance and density. Moreover, it ought to be noted that different elements identified with weight – like expanded stomach fat and diabetes – likewise have overall better bones and extended events of break. In this way, definite conclusions on the impact of a

Ketogenic diet on the bone thickness of these people can't be made.

Headaches are also one of the common symptoms experienced during the process of a Ketogenic diet. While your body is adjusting to ketosis, migraines can show for different reasons. You might likewise feel somewhat discombobulated and might encounter some influenza – like manifestations for a couple of days.

Constipation

Another common symptom of conducting low carb diet is constipation. It is typically a component of lack of hydration, salt misfortune, eating an excessive amount of dairy or an excess of nuts, or conceivably magnesium imbalances. All this causes issues with your digestion system.

Hypoglycemia (Low Blood Sugar)

Low blood sugar is another disadvantage for a person who has been eating a higher carb diet; their body is accustomed to putting out a precise measure of insulin to deal with the sugar which gets made from all that starch admission. Hence, when individuals consuming high carb food shifts to low carb diet, this sudden drop in carb access on a Ketogenic diet arrangement, might result in some short low glucose scenes that will feel frightening for an individual.

Chapter 4 – Ketogenic Diet Plan

Initiating the Ketogenic diet plan requires specific conditions that a person who is planning to start this diet plan has to consider. One of them is that before starting the low carb diet, one needs to consult with the physician or doctor to get the proper guideline. Low carb diet has many positive effects, but it also has an adverse impact as well on an individual's health. These especially effects those who have some issues such as heart problems, kidney problems, etc. therefore proper consultation from the doctor is required to have set of guideline what a person should intake and how do they need to start their diet plan.

Ketogenic diet plan duration varies from person to person and from the need as well. The term of this diet plan could be three days, one week, two weeks, one month or up to six months as well. An individual needs to follow the instructions given by the consultant, and they have to maintain a proper routine to monitor the diet. It means that while going to Ketogenic diet individual needs to consume only that food, that just contains low carbohydrate and have to abstain themselves from high calories, high carb food. People who previously consume a significant amount of sugar tends to start this process at a slow pace so that their body becomes used to the low sugar and later with time they can increase their intake of low carb food.

Setting-Up the Diet

To set the eating routine up, first an individual have to take their incline body weight and duplicate it by one. This will be the aggregate number of grams of protein they are required to eat every day. After with this, they would get this figure, various it by 4 (what number of calories are in one gram of protein) to get their aggregate calories originating from protein.

Presently whatever is left of their day by day necessity will arise from fat calories. Identifying sugar grams is not, particularly because as matter, of course, you will probably achieve your 30-50 grams for each day virtually by including green vegetables and the coincidental carbs that originate from your fat and protein sources.

To make sense of what number of fat grams particularly an individual needs, they would take the aggregate amount of calories it takes to keep up their body weight (ordinarily around 14-16 calories for every pound of body weight). Subtract their protein calories from that number and after that division by 9 (number of calories per gram of fat). This ought to give them the number of total fat grams they have to eat every day. Divide these figures by however numerous dinners they wish to cat every day to get the key format for their eating regimen. Also, make sure to devour a lot of fresh green vegetables for cell reinforcement and vitamin security, and you are ready to get started.

Weekend Carb Load

Presently this conveys us to the weekend carb load period and the "fun" part of general people. You are currently prepared to eat vast amounts of starch-containing nourishments, oat, bagels, rice chips, confection, pasta thus on are all great alternatives here. Since you won't be eating all that much fat by any means, there is more outlandish of a chance that these starches will get transformed into the muscle to fat quotients as they will be going towards topping off your muscle glycogen stores.

Many people will start their carb-up on Friday night and end it before bed on Saturday. This usually is most helpful as it's the point at which they are off of work and can unwind and appreciate the procedure. On the off chance that they aren't excessively worried about fat misfortune and are merely utilizing this eating regimen as an approach to keep up glucose levels, they can likely eat whatever starch nourishments they like amid this period. On the off chance that they have agonized over fast pick up, however, then they require the math.

Attempt and mean to keep their protein the same at one gram for every pound of body weight and after that take in 10-12 grams of starches for each kilogram of body weight. Begin making these starches (ordinarily the main piece in fluid-structure) directly after your keep going workout on Friday night. This is the point at which their body is ready to rock and roll to uptake the starches, and it will be most helpful to you.

Note that people typically can have some fat here, since it will be challenging to devour a large number of the sustenance they genuinely need to eat without being permitted any (pizza for occurrence). They do their best to keep your fat grams around their body weight in kilograms (so on the off chance that person measure 80 kg's, eat close to 80 grams of fat).

On a second note, a few people discover they jump at the chance to eat a little organic product alongside protein before their last workout on Friday night as this will restore their liver glycogen levels and give them the vitality they have to push through that workout. Besides, by refilling the liver glycogen, they will put their body into a somewhat more anabolic state, so they don't see as much vitality breakdown.

How to Get Start with Ketogenic Diet?

While starting the Ketogenic plan, certain conditions need to be considered. One of them is that not everyone can follow the Ketogenic diet plan. Different people based on their age, health, and other conditions have different diet plans recommended by experts. However, people who should not follow Ketogenic diet are:

1. Individuals with gallbladder malady or without a gallbladder, since fat is harder to process;

2. Individuals who have had bariatric surgery (weight reduction/gastric detour) since fats are more difficult to ingest;

3. Individuals with an individual metabolic issue that meddle with typical fat digestion system;

4. Ladies who are pregnant or breastfeeding, because protein necessities are higher;

5. Kids, since protein needs shift by age hence children should not undertake this diet plan;

6. Individuals with pancreatic inadequacy, since fats are harder to process;

7. individuals inclined to kidney stones (maybe because of salt and liquid equalization changes); and

8. Individuals who are thin (BMI of 20 or less) because weight reduction might happen for a few (extra fat calories might be required).

All these kind of people should not start with Ketogenic diet plan since there are various side-effects that they might be experienced due to a Ketogenic diet. For grown-ups taking a Ketogenic diet, the most widely recognized entanglements incorporate weight reduction, blockage, the risk of bone fracture, an increase in thirst level, consistent urination, frequent mood swings and expanded levels of cholesterol and triglycerides. Ladies might likewise encounter amenorrhea or different disturbances to the menstrual cycle. Therefore, all these factors need to be considered before starting up with a Ketogenic diet plan.

Chapter 5 – Foods To Apply Ketosis Diet

Before understanding the type of foods to undertake during the Ketogenic diet, it is essential that an individual must consider how much calories or food he or she must intake per day. With the help of ideal body weight, BMI or other calorie counts a person can identify how many calories he or she must take on a daily basis so that they can achieve their target weight. There have been various applications introduced that people can install in their phones and through those applications, they can obtain their information that includes their current weight, gender, age and ideal weight that they want to get.

By taking this information, these applications tell the person how many calories they must take on a daily basis to reach their ideal weight. And through these applications and perfect body weight, individuals need to identify their regular proportion of fat, protein, carbohydrate incorrect grams and calorie portion for better understanding and following the diet plan. The foods that should be undertaken during Ketogenic Diet includes:

Fats and Oils

- Fats will be the significant share of a day by day calorie admission when individuals are on a Ketogenic diet, so decisions ought to be made considering their assimilation framework. One needs to have a harmony between their Omega-3's and Omega-6's, so eating things like wild salmon, fish, trout, and shellfish can give an adjusted eating routine of Omega-3's
- Soaked and monounsaturated fats, for example, margarine, macadamia nuts, avocado, egg yolks,

and coconut oil are all the more artificially steady and less provocative to a great many people, so they are favored.

- Foods that are high in fats and oils include Avocado, beef tallow, butter, chicken fat, non-hydrated lard. Other foods include macadamia nuts, and mayonnaise is also high in fat, olive oil, coconut oil & butter, red palm oil and peanut butter
- Fats and oils can be consolidated in various diverse approaches to add to your suppers – sauces, dressings, or simply basic garnish off a bit of meat with butter.

Protein

- Ideally eating anything that is gotten wild like catfish, cod, salmon or snapper, trout, and fish.
- Shellfish: Shellfishes, clams, lobster, crab, scallops, mussels, and squid.
- Entire Eggs: Try to purchase them from a nearby market if conceivable. People can set them up in

various diverse ways like fricasseed, deviled, bubbled, poached, and mixed.

- Meat: Hamburger, Veal, Goat, Sheep, and another wild diversion. Grass sustained is favored as it has a superior unsaturated fat number.
- Pork: Pork loin and ham. Be careful of included sugars in ham.
- Poultry: Chicken, Duck, Quail, Bird. Unfenced or natural is an optimal decision here if.
- Bacon and Wiener: Check marks for anything cured in sugar, or on the off chance that it contains fillers.
- Nutty spread: Go for the typical nutty spread; however be cautious as they have high numbers of Omega-6's and starches. Attempt to select macadamia nut margarine on the off chance that they can.

Vegetables

- Vegetables are considered healthy. Hence, people on a Ketogenic diet are more encouraged to increase their intake of vegetables that are taken from the ground and are green.

Nuts and Seeds

- Nuts and seeds are best when they are simmered to evacuate any hostile to supplements. Attempt to maintain a critical distance from peanuts if conceivable, as they are vegetables which are not exceptionally allowed on the Ketogenic diet nourishment list.
- Macadamias, walnuts, and almonds are one of the best as far as your carbs include and can be eaten little sums.

- Cashews and pistachios are higher in carbs, so ensure you measure these deliberately. Nuts are high in Omega-6 Unsaturated fats, so attempt to be cautious with overutilization. Nut and seed flours, for example, almond flour and processed flaxseed are extraordinary to substitute for normal flour. This implies preparing should be possible with some restraint.

The following chart properly explains the food that a person is undertaking Ketogenic diet must consider in his or her diet plan to reduce their weight in the short term.

Beverages

Drinks that it must include in their diet plan are water, tea, coffee, and spirits. Drinks like water should frequently be consumed whereas tea and coffees intake should be moderately done and for spirits and wines, their consumption should be occasionally or rarely but not frequently. Water is crucial as many people face the issue of dehydration. Therefore, six to eight glasses of water is recommended.

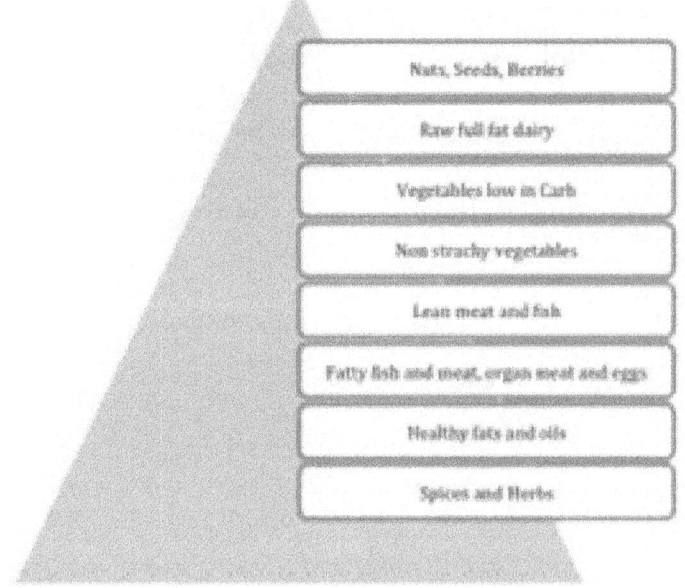

Sweeteners

Avoiding anything sweet is, by and large, the best wagered – it will control yearnings to a minimal level, which advances accomplishment on the Ketogenic diet. On the off chance that you need to have something sweet, however, pick an artificial sweetener. Attempt to follow fluid sweeteners as they don't have included covers, for example, maltodextrin and dextrose which have carbs. Stevia, a liquid structure is favored Sucralose, a fluid composition is supported, Erythritol, Xylitol, Friar Natural product, Agave Nectar. All these kinds of sweeteners must be considered to reduce the cravings of having something sweet.

Chapter 6 – Ketogenic Diet Mistakes and Tips

There are several common mistakes that individuals commit while being on Ketogenic diet and many of them are featured below.

Increase the Intake of Protein

Many people raise their level of protein because protein is something that might increase the glucose level as well. Moreover, Ketogenic diet is meant to control the glucose level if more protein is added to the routine, it would mean more glucose. In other words, the goal will not be possible to be achieved.

Not Eating Enough Fat

We have been adapted to keep away from fats, and it doesn't feel right to devour more. Sugar and grains can bring about glucose to rise and causes the body to store fat. Eating fat permits your body to smolder fat and get incline. Decreasing carbs allow your body to blaze what is left, and that is fat.

Not Eating Enough Sodium in Eating Regimen

A low carb Ketogenic diet causes the body to discharge sodium in the body. It is one reason that a man loses 5+ lbs. in the first week; it is for the most part water weight at first. It is additionally the motivation behind why a few individuals feel hopeless the first couple of days and has migraines, sickness, weariness and woozy side effects.

Eating stock with salt and adding salt to your nourishment assists with this and makes your side effects disappear quicker. When you alter you begin feeling decent on this eating regimen as your body modifies.

Exercises to conduct during your diet

Specific exercises are recommended during Ketogenic diet that an individual must undertake such as callisthenic exercise that does not include any machinery or any instruments all it requires human movements, for example, pushups, incline pushups, chin-ups, squats, straight leg deadlift, abdominals, etc.

Chapter 7 – Ketogenic Recipes

Snacks

For snacks, smoothies are recommended, such as creamy chocolate milk, which would include unsweetened almond milk, one packet artificial sweetener, heavy cream, chocolate powder and crushed ice. All these ingredients must be blended and then served.

Drinks

- Water: you be drinking at least a gallon of water a day. As long as this requirement is met, then other things are fair game.
- Diet soda: now you must be careful, the artificial sweetener can kick you out of ketosis. So limit it to one per day.
- Diet soda + 2 Tbsp cream
- Almond milk
- Green tea

- Black Tea
- Water: yes, I'm mentioning it again. (It's that important).

Peanut butter and Cacao Protein shake

Ingredients

- 2 cups almond milk
- 4/5 ice cubes
- 1 scoop vanilla whey protein
- 2 spoonfuls of peanut-butter
- 1 tbs of baking cocoa

Instructions

Blend well and then you now have a delicious chocolate vanilla peanut butter shake, packed with protein and fat, but only about 10g carbs! This recipe is highly modifiable, take out the PB and lower the carb total.

Breakfast

For breakfast, it is recommended that low carb fruit must be undertaken in the morning. In this recipe all fruit containing low carb must be included together and if required heavy cream must be added. Fruits may include fresh strawberries, raw raspberries, peaches, avocado, apricot, etc.

Breakfast Meal #1 - Cinnamon Protein Waffles

Ingredients

For Waffles:

- 1/2 cup (62 g) whole-wheat flour
- 2/3 scoop (22 g) MusclePharm Cinnamon Bun Combat Powder
- 1 teaspoon of granulated Erythritol
- 1/2 teaspoon of cinnamon
- 1/4 teaspoon of baking powder
- 1/4 cup + 2 teaspoons of unsweetened almond milk
- 1 whole large egg

- 1/4 cup canned pumpkin, not pie filling (see notes below for subs)
- 1/2 teaspoon of vanilla extract

For Cream Cheese Icing:

- 1/4 cup plain nonfat Greek yogurt
- 2 teaspoon of reduced fat cream cheese
- 1 teaspoon granulated Stevia or erythritol

Instructions

1. Preheat waffle iron to medium heat in the oven. Mix all the ingredients together. Flour, protein powder, baking powder, and cinnamon in the bowl.
2. In another bowl, mix the eggs, almond milk, and vanilla extract.
3. Add wet ingredients to dry and gently mix until combined. Spray the iron with cooking spray.

4. Spoon batter into the waffle iron to make three separate waffles. Cook for a few minutes until the colours turn golden brown.
5. Mix the cream cheese and the yogurt and Stevia together. Spoon icing into a plastic bag. Grab a scissor or knife and cut off the end portion off and pump out the frosting onto your waffles.
6. Sprinkle some cinnamon and bonne appetite!

Breakfast Meal #2 - Ketogenic Low Carb Pancakes:

Ingredients

- 5 large eggs (keto version: 2 whole egg + 8 yolks) 50 grams of desiccated coconut, ground to flour
- 50 grams of hazelnuts, ground to flour
- Use a small piece of butter or coconut oil for frying
- 1 level tablespoon mixed spice

Instructions

1. Grind up the coconut and chopped hazels (I use a coffee grinder).
2. Mix them together with the mixed spice in a bowl.
3. Beat the eggs in another bowl.
4. Beat in the ground nuts until they make a batter with a smooth consistency.

5. Melt knob of butter or coconut oil in a hot frying pan then pour in about 1/4 of the batter to cover the base thinly.
6. Turn once with a wide spatula.
7. Place on a plate in a warm oven while you cook the others.
8. Serve with clotted cream, or whatever suits your version of this now versatile recipe.

Breakfast Meal #3 - Microwave Flax Muffins:

Ingredients

- 1 egg
- 1 splash of heavy whipping cream
- 1 to 2 teaspoons of nay sweetener of your choice
- 1 pinch salt
- 1 teaspoon of vanilla extract
- 4 teaspoon of ground flax meal
- (Sometimes I add 1 teaspoon or so of unsweetened cocoa powder to make it taste like a brownie)

Instructions

1. Mix in a microwave safe bowl and microwave for 1 to 1 and a half minutes.
2. If it gets too dry, plop a pat of butter on top of the finished muffin and let it melt in.

Main Course

#1 - Low Carb Pizza:

Ingredients

For the main course, low carb pizza is recommended. Low carb pizza contains olive oil, extensive head natural cauliflower, trimmed and cleaved into little pieces, white onion minced, margarine, water, eggs destroyed mozzarella cheddar, fennel seed, Italian flavoring, parmesan, Home-style Pizza sauce (it's the most reduced in carb), and Italian wiener (check carb number, ought to be under 1 for each ounce)

Instructions

- Preheat the stove to 450F. Oil a 17 x 11 treat sheet with olive oil.
- In a substantial skillet with a cover, liquefy the spread and include the onion and cauliflower. Sauté the vegetables over low to medium warmth until the cauliflower is verging on done.

- Include the water. Cover and steam until the cauliflower is utterly delicate. Expel from warmth, exchange to a glass or clay dish to cool.

- While cauliflower is cooling, add the Italian wiener to the skillet and cook until done, separating it into little pieces with a spatula. Expel the frankfurter from the skillet and channel on paper towels to uproot overabundance fat. Put aside to cool.

- When cauliflower has cooled down, allot three containers and spot in a sustenance processor. Process it to smooth consistency. Scratch the pureed cauliflower into a blending dish. Include the eggs, minced mozzarella cheddar, flavors and parmesan cheddar to the cauliflower. Blend well. Utilizing a spatula, spread the cauliflower mixture on the lubed treat sheet. Attempt to spread it out with the goal that it is an even thickness everywhere.

- Prepare the outside layer at 450F for around 20 minutes, or until the surface looks cooked and its chestnut around edges.

- While the low-carb pizza covering is heating, cleave up the cooked wiener into better pieces (you can simply spin it in the sustenance processor for a few seconds).
- Pour the container of Ragu sauce in a little pot, and include the hacked Italian hot dog. Cover and convey to a moderate stew over low to medium warmth.
- At the point when the hull is done, take it out of the stove, and switch broiler setting to sear. Stove rack ought to be around 4 inches from the grill.
- Pour the sauce and hotdog blend over the highest point of the hull, and spread around with a spatula. (It will be a dainty covering).
- Spread the covering and sauce uniformly with the Italian cheddar mix.
- Put the low carb pizza back in the stove, and cook until cheddar melts and starts to air pocket and cocoa.
- Expel from the stove, cut into 12 cuts with a pizza cutter.
- Serve and Appreciate!

#2 - California Chicken Omelette:

Ingredients

- 2 eggs
- 2 slices of bacon
- 1 ounce of deli cut chicken
- 1/4 avocado
- 1 Campari tomato
- 1 tablespoon of mayo
- 1 teaspoon of mustard

Instructions

1. Crack 2 eggs in a bowl and then add them to a hot pan. Pull the sides of the eggs towards the center to cook the omelette a bit faster.
2. Season with salt and pepper.
3. Once your eggs are thoroughly cooked (about 5 minutes), add your chicken, bacon and avocado and tomatoes. You can also add a tablespoon of mayo and a bit of mustard.

4. Fold the omelette over onto itself and cover with a lid. Cook for an extra 5 minutes after.
5. Once the eggs are cooked and everything is warm inside, you're
6. Ready to eat. Enjoy!

#3 - Avocado Egg Salad:

Ingredients

- 4 large eggs, free-range or organic
- 1 large avocado
- 4 cups mixed lettuce such as lamb lettuce, arugula, etc.
- ½ cup soured cream *or* full-fat yogurt (115 g / 4.1 ounces) *or* ¼ cup mayonnaise
- 2 cloves garlic, crushed
- 1 tomato
- 2 teaspoon Dijon mustard
- salt and pepper to taste
- *Optional:* chives, fresh herbs and extra virgin olive oil for garnish.

Instructions

1. Start by cooking the eggs. Fill a small saucepan with water up to three quarters. Wait till the eggs begin to boil. Using a spoon or hand, dip each egg in and out of the boiling water. Wait approximately 10 minutes

before they boil. When done, remove from the heat and place the eggs in a bowl of cold water. When the eggs are chilled, peel off the shells. You can make the dressing by mixing together the soured cream, crushed garlic and mustard. You can also add salt and pepper for extra taste.

2. Wash and drain the greens in a salad spinner or just by pat drying using a paper towel. Place the greens in a bowl and mix all the ingredients with the dressing. Halve, deseed, peel and slice the avocado and place on top of the greens.

3. Add the quartered eggs and you can also season with more salt and pepper to taste.

Final Words

Thank you again for purchasing this book! I really hope this book is able to help you.

The next step is for you to join our email newsletter to receive updates on any upcoming new book releases or promotions. You can sign-up for free and as a bonus, you will also receive our "*7 Fitness Mistakes You Don't Know You're Making*" book! This bonus book breaks down many of the most common fitness mistakes and will demystify many of the complexities and science of getting into shape. Having all this fitness knowledge and science organized into an actionable step-by-step book will help you get started in the right direction in your fitness journey! To join our free email newsletter and grab your free book, please visit the link and signup: www.hmwpublishing.com/gift

Finally, if you enjoyed this book, then I would like to ask you for a favor, would you be kind enough to leave a review for this book? It would be greatly appreciated!

Thank you and good luck in your journey!

About the Co-Author

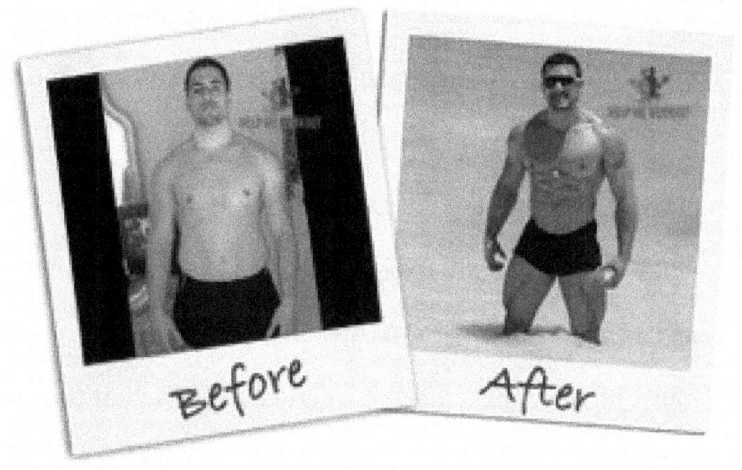

My name is George Kaplo; I'm a certified personal trainer from Montreal, Canada. I'll start off by saying I'm not the biggest guy you will ever meet and this has never really been my goal. In fact, I started working out to overcome my biggest insecurity when I was younger, which was my self-confidence. This was due to my height measuring only 5 foot 5 inches (168cm), it pushed me down to attempt anything I ever wanted to achieve in life. You may be going through some challenges right now, or you may simply want to get fit, and I can certainly relate.

For me personally, I was always kind of interested in the health & fitness world and wanted to gain some muscle due to the numerous bullying in my teenage years about my height and my overweight body. I figured I couldn't do anything about my height, but I sure can do something about how my body looked like. This was the beginning of my transformation journey. I had no idea where to start, but I just got started. I felt worried and afraid at times that other people would make fun of me for doing the exercises the wrong way. I always wished I had a friend that was next to me who was knowledgeable enough to help me get started and "show me the ropes."

After a lot of work, studying and countless trial and errors. Some people began to notice how I was getting more fit and how I was starting to form a keen interest in the topic. This led many friends and new faces to come to me and ask me for fitness advice. At first, it seemed odd when people asked me to help them get in shape. But what kept me going is when they started to see changes in their own body and told me it's the first time that they saw real results!

From there, more people kept coming to me, and it made me realize after so much reading and studying in this field that it did help me but it also allowed me to help others. I'm now a fully certified personal trainer and have trained numerous clients to date who have achieved amazing results.

Today, my brother Alex Kaplo (also a Certified Personal Trainer) and I own & operate this publishing venture, where we bring passionate and expert authors to write about health and fitness topics. We also run an online fitness website "HelpMeWorkout.com" and I would love to connect with by inviting you to visit the website on the following page and signing up to our e-mail newsletter (you will even get a free book).

Last but not least, if you are in the position I was once in and you want some guidance, don't hesitate and ask... I'll be there to help you out!

Your friend and coach,

George Kaplo
Certified Personal Trainer

Download another book for Free

I want to thank you for purchasing this book and offer you another book (just as long and valuable as this book), "Health & Fitness Mistakes You Don't Know You're Making", completely free.

Visit the link below to signup and receive it:

www.hmwpublishing.com/gift

In this book, I will break down the most common health & fitness mistakes, you are probably committing right now, and I will reveal how you can easily get in the best shape of your life!

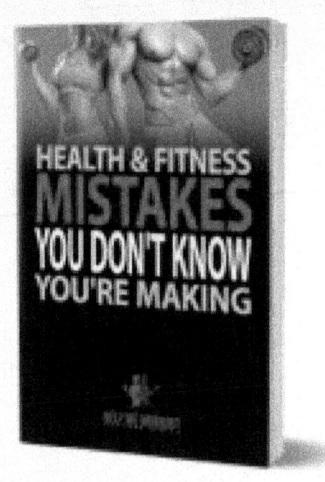

In addition to this valuable gift, you will also have an opportunity to get our new books for free, enter giveaways, and receive other valuable emails from me. Again, visit the link to sign up:

www.hmwpublishing.com/gift

Copyright 2017 by HMW Publishing - All Rights Reserved.

This document by HMW Publishing owned by the A&G Direct Inc company, is geared towards providing exact and reliable information in regards to the topic and issue covered. The publication is sold with the idea that the publisher is not required to render accounting, officially permitted, or otherwise, qualified services. If advice is necessary, legal or professional, a practiced individual in the profession should be ordered.

From a Declaration of Principles which was accepted and approved equally by a Committee of the American Bar Association and a Committee of Publishers and Associations.

In no way is it legal to reproduce, duplicate, or transmit any part of this document in either electronic means or in printed format. Recording of this publication is strictly prohibited, and any storage of this document is not allowed unless with written permission from the publisher. All rights reserved.

The information provided herein is stated to be truthful and consistent, in that any liability, in terms of inattention or otherwise, by any usage or abuse of any policies, processes, or directions contained within is the solitary and utter responsibility of the recipient reader. Under no circumstances will any legal responsibility or blame be held against the publisher for any reparation, damages, or monetary loss due to the information herein, either directly or indirectly.

The information herein is offered for informational purposes solely, and is universal as so. The presentation of the information is without contract or any type of guarantee assurance.

The trademarks that are used are without any consent, and the publication of the trademark is without permission or backing by the trademark owner. All trademarks and brands within this book are for clarifying purposes only and are the owned by the owners themselves, not affiliated with this document.

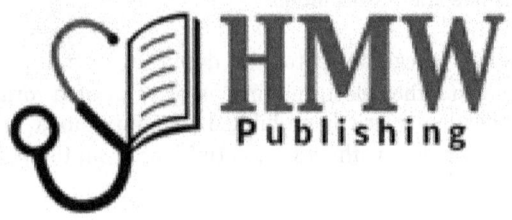

For more great books visit:

HMWPublishing.com

www.ingramcontent.com/pod-product-compliance
Lightning Source LLC
Chambersburg PA
CBHW071123030426
42336CB00013BA/2184